KETO DIET COOKBOOK

The best recipes on the ketogenic diet to lose weight. Burn fat and increase your metabolism easily by changing your lifestyle by eating healthy and low-carb and low-calorie foods.

LIFESTYLE KETO

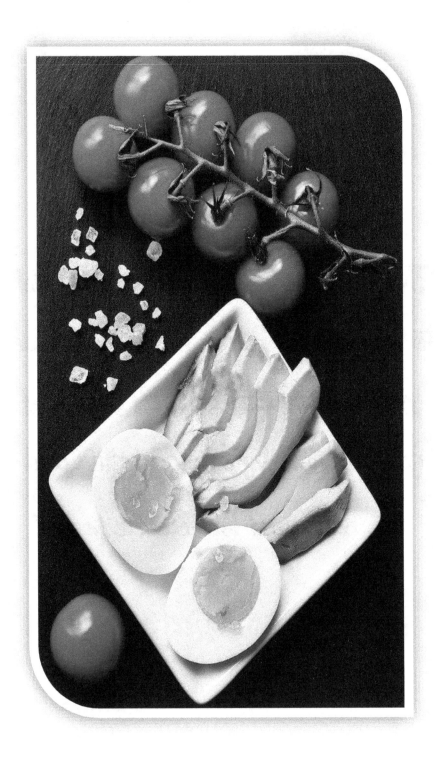

that may befall them after undertaking information described herein.

Additionally, the information in the following pages is intended only for informational purposes and should thus be thought of as universal. As befitting its nature, it is presented without assurance regarding its prolonged validity or interim quality. Trademarks that are mentioned are done without written consent and can in no way be considered an endorsement from the trademark holder.

Table of Contents

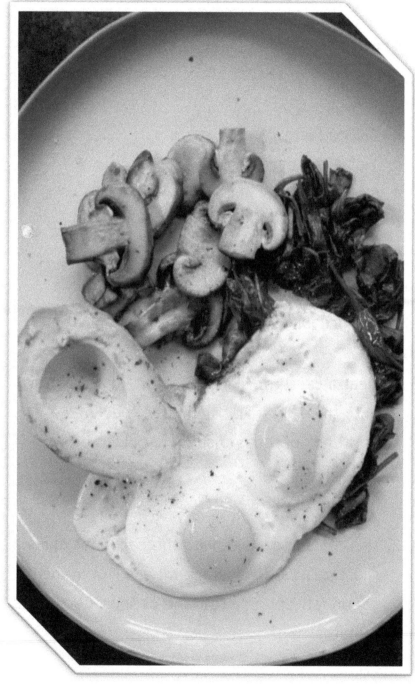

1. Classic Bacon & Eggs

Ingredients

- ❖ 2 large eggs
- ❖ Salt to taste
- ❖ 1 pinch of pepper
- ❖ 8 pieces of bacon slices
- ❖ 4 cherry tomatoes
- ❖ 1 teaspoon chopped cilantro

Instructions

1. Heat a cast-iron skillet. Place the bacon slices onto the skillet. Fry them on a medium flame until they become crispy and golden brown. Take them out.

2. Use the same skillet with the bacon fat to cook the eggs. Carefully crack the eggs onto the bacon fat. Sprinkle salt and pepper. Cook for 2 minutes.

3. Serve eggs and bacon with cherry tomato and
   cilantro.

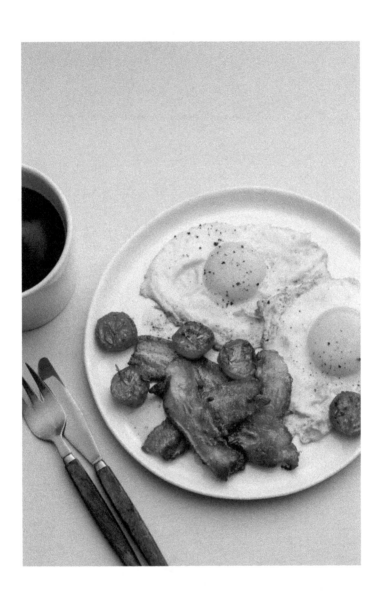

2. Poached egg with Spinach Stir Fry

Ingredients

- ❖ 1 egg
- ❖ 1 tablespoon butter
- ❖ Salt to taste
- ❖ 1 tablespoon sunflower oil
- ❖ 1 cup chopped spinach
- ❖ ½ teaspoon black salt
- ❖ 2 tablespoon heavy cream
- ❖ 1 teaspoon pepper

Instructions

1. Heat butter into a frying pan. Carefully crack an egg. Sprinkle some salt. Cook for 2 minutes. Take it out from the frying pan.

2. Add sunflower oil into the same pan. Add spinach, black salt, and pepper. Sautee for 5 minutes.

3. Place fried egg and spinach onto a serving plate. Serve with a dollop of heavy cream.

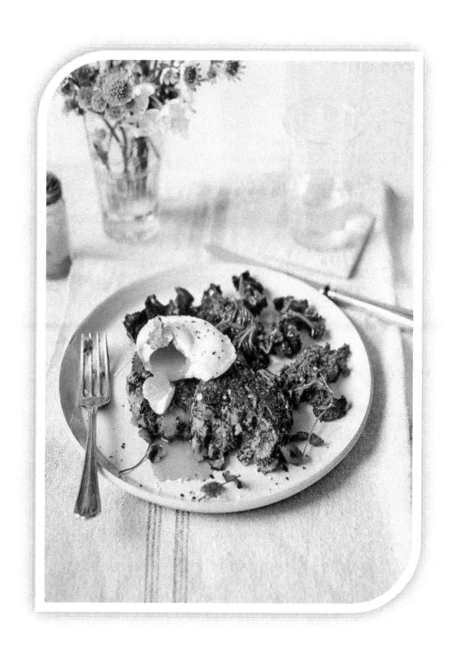

3. Spinach Scrambled Egg

Ingredients

- ❖ 2 large eggs
- ❖ 4 tablespoon heavy cream
- ❖ 2 tablespoon butter
- ❖ 2 large onion, sliced
- ❖ Salt to taste
- ❖ 1 teaspoon pepper
- ❖ 1 cup chopped spinach

Instructions

1. Take a mixing bowl and add egg, heavy cream, salt, and pepper. Mix well.

2. Melt butter into a frying pan. Sautee onion and spinach for 5 minutes. Add the beaten egg mixture.

3. Stir constantly to mix everything. Cook for 4 to 5 minutes.

4. Serve.

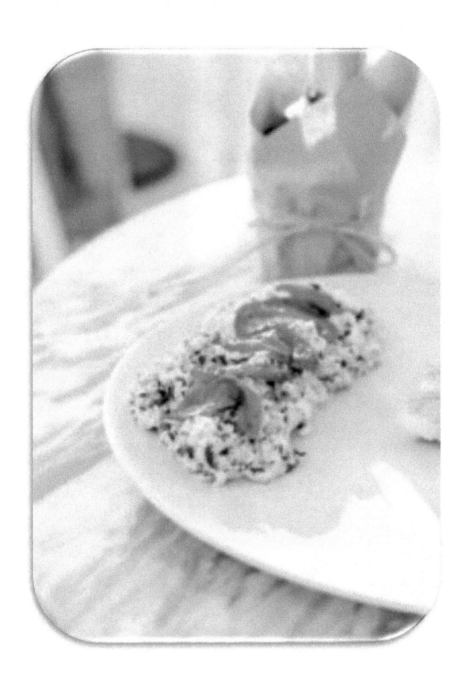

4. Bacon Pancake

Ingredients

- ❖ 2 large eggs
- ❖ ¼ cup almond flour
- ❖ ¼ cup grated cottage cheese
- ❖ 2 tablespoon heavy cream
- ❖ ¼ cup bacon, cooked and crumbled
- ❖ Salt to taste
- ❖ 1 teaspoon pepper
- ❖ ½ teaspoon cumin powder
- ❖ 1 tablespoon lemon juice
- ❖ Butter to brush the frying pan

Instructions

1. Take all the ingredients into a food processor. Make a smooth batter.

2. Brush the frying pan with butter. Add ¼ cup pancake batter. Spread evenly. Cook on a

medium flame for 4 minutes. Flip and cook for another 4 minutes. Do the same with the remaining batter.

3. Serve.

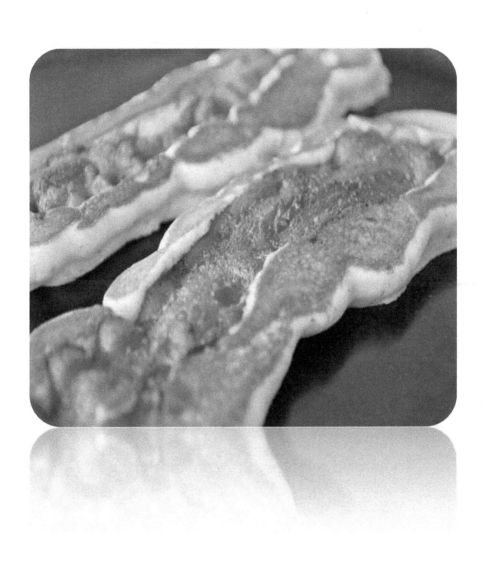

5. Classic Scrambled Egg

Ingredients

- ❖ 1 tablespoon butter
- ❖ 2 large eggs
- ❖ Salt to taste
- ❖ ½ teaspoon pepper

Instructions

1. Take a mixing bowl and add eggs, salt, and pepper. Mix well.

2. Melt butter into a frying pan. Add the egg mixture.
   Cook for 5 minutes. Stir constantly.

3. Serve.

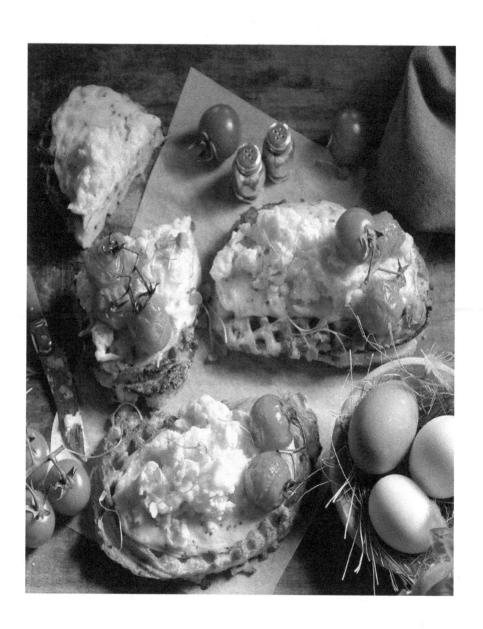

6. Spinach Frittata

Ingredients

- ❖ 3 eggs
- ❖ 1 cup chopped spinach
- ❖ 1 tablespoon onion slices
- ❖ 4 tablespoons grated cheddar cheese
- ❖ ¼ cup heavy cream
- ❖ Salt to taste
- ❖ 1 teaspoon pepper
- ❖ 1 tablespoon chopped dill

Ingredients

1. Preheat the oven to 350F. Grease a baking dish with butter.

2. Add eggs into a mixing bowl. Beat well. Add all the other ingredients and mix perfectly.

3. Pour the mixture into the baking dish. Bake for 30 minutes.

4. Serve.

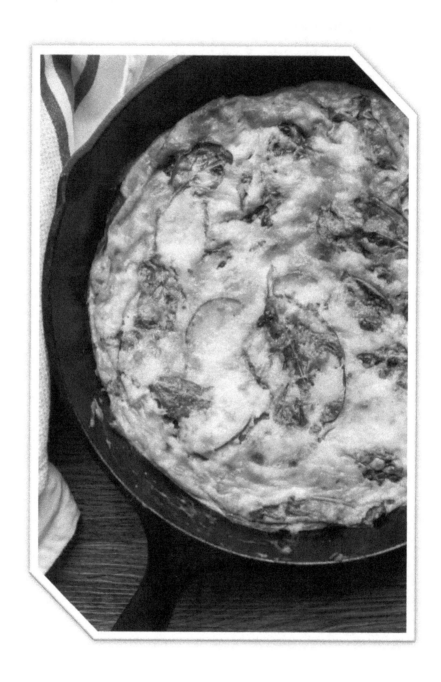

7. Apple Peanut Butter Chia Pudding

Ingredients

- ❖ 1 cup peanut milk
- ❖ 1 tablespoon peanut butter
- ❖ ½ teaspoon vanilla extract
- ❖ 2 tablespoon chia seeds
- ❖ 1 teaspoon stevia
- ❖ ¼ cup chopped apple

Instructions

1. Mix peanut milk, peanut butter, vanilla extract, stevia, and chia seeds into a mixing bowl. Put it in the refrigerator for 4 hours.

2. Top with chopped apple. Serve.

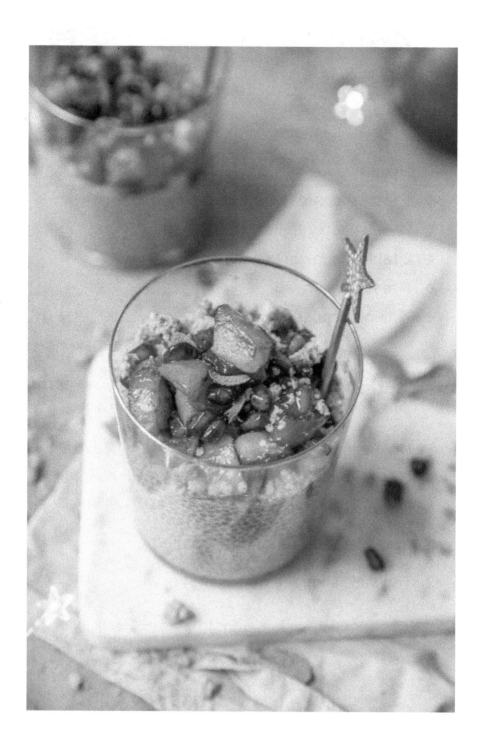

8. Cheese Omelet

Ingredients

- ❖ 2 large eggs
- ❖ 2 tablespoons grated mozzarella cheese
- ❖ 2 tablespoons grated parmesan cheese
- ❖ 2 tablespoons grated cheddar cheese
- ❖ 2 tablespoons grated cottage cheese
- ❖ 2 tablespoons cream cheese
- ❖ Salt to taste
- ❖ 1 teaspoon pepper
- ❖ 2 tablespoon butter

Instructions

1. Take a mixing bowl and add eggs, mozzarella cheese, cream cheese, cheddar cheese, parmesan cheese, salt, and pepper. Mix nicely.

2. Melt butter into a frying pan. Pour the egg mixture and spread evenly. Cover with the lid.

Cook on a low flame for 5 minutes. Then flip carefully and cook for another 5 minutes.

3. Serve.

Keto Lunch

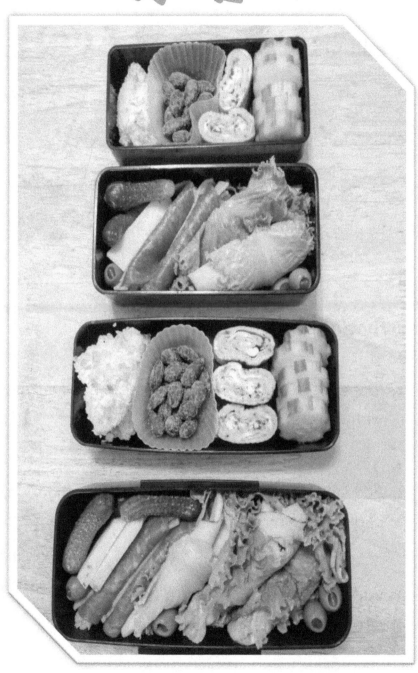

1. Broccoli Steak

Ingredients

- ❖ 1 broccoli
- ❖ Salt to taste
- ❖ 1 teaspoon paprika
- ❖ 1 tablespoon butter
- ❖ 1 tablespoon olive oil
- ❖ 1 tablespoon ginger-garlic paste

Instructions

1. Preheat the oven to 400F. Grease a baking tray with cooking oil.

2. Add salt, pepper, butter, olive oil, and ginger-garlic paste into a mixing bowl. Mix well.

3. Cut the Broccoli into ½-inch thick steaks. Add into the mixture and rub well.

4. Place the broccoli steaks onto the baking tray. Bake for 25 minutes.

5. Serve.

2. Stir-Fried Bottle Gourd

Ingredients

- ❖ 2 tablespoons sunflower oil
- ❖ 2 large onion, sliced
- ❖ 1 teaspoon minced garlic
- ❖ 1 teaspoon grated ginger
- ❖ 2 chopped green chilies
- ❖ ½ teaspoon turmeric powder
- ❖ 1 teaspoon·cumin powder
- ❖ Salt to taste
- ❖ 1 cup finely sliced bottle gourd

Instructions

1. Heat sunflower oil into a frying pan. Add onion, garlic, ginger, and chili. Sautee for 3 minutes.

2. Now add the bottle gourd. Sprinkle salt, turmeric powder, and cumin powder. Stir fry on a medium flame for 10 to 15 minutes.

3. Serve.

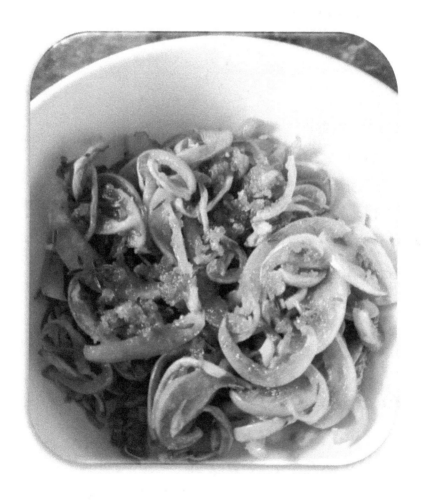

3. Tilapia in Tomato Gravy

Ingredients

- ❖ 4 tilapia fillets
- ❖ 2 onion
- ❖ 4 cloves of garlic
- ❖ 3 tomato
- ❖ 2 red chili
- ❖ 1 tablespoon lemon juice
- ❖ 1 teaspoon cumin powder
- ❖ ½ teaspoon turmeric powder
- ❖ 2 tablespoon cilantro
- ❖ Salt to taste
- ❖ 2 tablespoon extra-virgin olive oil
- ❖ 1.4 cup of water

Instructions

1. Take a food processor. Add tomato, onion, garlic, red chili, lemon juice, cumin powder, turmeric powder, salt, and cilantro. Make a fine paste.

2. Heat olive oil into a saucepan. Add the spice mix. Cook for 5 minutes.

3. Add the water. Let it come to a boil.

4. Now carefully add the tilapia fillets. Cook on a low flame for 15 minutes.

5. Serve.

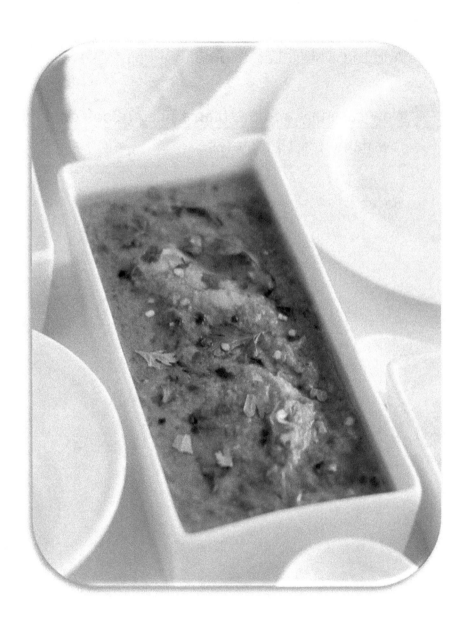

4. Pumpkin in Mustard Gravy

Ingredients

- ❖ 1 cup pumpkin, cut into cubes
- ❖ 2 tablespoons mustard oil
- ❖ 2 tablespoons onion paste
- ❖ 2 teaspoons ginger-garlic paste
- ❖ 4 tablespoons mustard paste
- ❖ Salt to taste
- ❖ ½ teaspoon turmeric powder
- ❖ 1 teaspoon red chili powder
- ❖ 1 teaspoon coriander powder
- ❖ 1 cup of water

Ingredients

1. Heat mustard oil into a saucepan. Add onion paste, ginger-garlic paste, turmeric powder, red chili powder, coriander powder, and mustard paste. Cook for 5 minutes.

2. Now add water and salt. Let it come to a boil.

3. Now add the pumpkin cubes. Cook on a low flame for 10 minutes.

4. Serve.

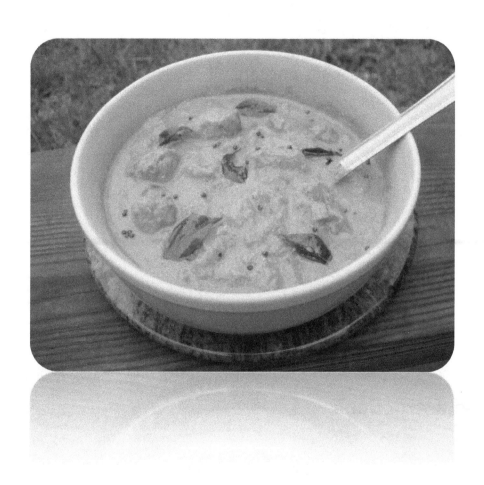

5. Salmon in Mustard Gravy

Ingredients

- ❖ 4 salmon fillets
- ❖ 3 tablespoons mustard oil
- ❖ ½ teaspoon whole mustard
- ❖ 2 tablespoons onion paste
- ❖ 2 teaspoons ginger-garlic paste
- ❖ 4 tablespoons mustard paste
- ❖ Salt to taste
- ❖ ½ teaspoon turmeric powder
- ❖ 1 teaspoon red chili powder
- ❖ 1 teaspoon cumin powder
- ❖ 1 cup of water

Instructions

1. Heat mustard oil. Add the whole mustard seeds. Fry for 30 seconds. It will start to lose a spicy aroma.

2. Now add onion paste, ginger-garlic paste, turmeric powder, red chili powder, cumin powder, and mustard paste. Cook for 5 minutes.

3. Add water and salt. Let it come to a boil. Add salmon fillets. Cook on a low flame for 15 minutes.

4. Serve.

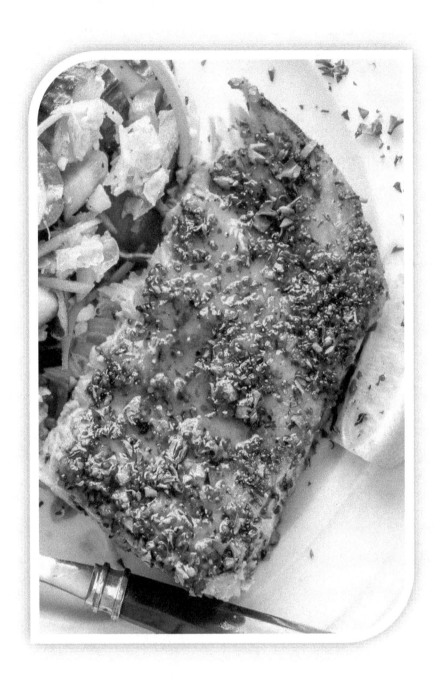

6. Stir-Fried Chicken

Ingredients

- ❖ 2 tablespoons sunflower oil
- ❖ 2 large onion, sliced
- ❖ 2 teaspoon minced garlic
- ❖ 1 teaspoon grated ginger
- ❖ 1 cup chicken, cut into small cube
- ❖ Salt to taste
- ❖ 1 teaspoon red chili powder
- ❖ 1 teaspoon Indian spice mix
- ❖ 2 teaspoon chopped cilantro

Instructions

1. Heat oil in a frying pan. Sautee onion, garlic, and ginger for 3 minutes.

2. Add chicken, salt, red chili powder, and Indian spice mix. Mix well. Fry for 12 minutes. Stir constantly.

3. Sprinkle cilantro. Cook for 2 minutes.

4. Serve.

7. Garlic Lemon Baked Cod

Ingredients

- ❖ 4 cod fillets
- ❖ 2 tablespoons butter
- ❖ 2 tablespoons lemon juice
- ❖ 2 teaspoons garlic powder
- ❖ 1 teaspoon pink salt
- ❖ 1 teaspoon pepper
- ❖ 1 teaspoon paprika

Instructions

1. Preheat the oven to 350F. Lightly grease a baking tray.

2. Add butter, lemon juice, garlic powder, pink salt, pepper, and paprika. Mix thoroughly.

3. Add cod fillets. Rub well. Marinate for 15 minutes.

4. Now bake the cod fillets for 15 minutes. Serve.

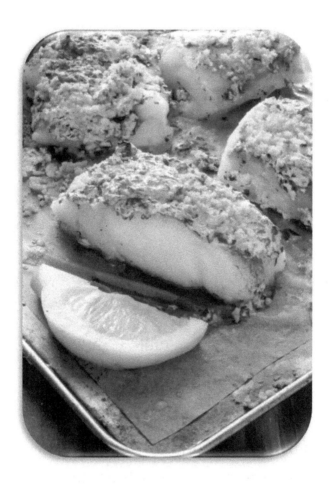

8. Roasted Cottage Cheese in Yogurt Gravy

Ingredients

- ❖ 1 cup cottage cheese cubes
- ❖ Salt to taste
- ❖ 1 teaspoon red chili powder
- ❖ 1 tablespoon sunflower oil
- ❖ 2 tablespoons butter
- ❖ 1 cup Greek yogurt
- ❖ 1 tablespoon garlic powder
- ❖ 1 teaspoon ginger powder
- ❖ ½ teaspoon stevia
- ❖ 1 teaspoon pepper

Instructions

1. Preheat the oven to 350F. Grease a baking dish with cooking spray.

2. Place the cottage cheese cubes onto the baking tray. Sprinkle oil, salt, and red chili powder. Bake for 10 minutes.

3. Add Greek yogurt, garlic powder, ginger powder, stevia, and pepper into a bowl. Mix well.

4. Melt butter into a saucepan. Add the yogurt sauce. Let it come to a boil.

5. Now add the cottage cheese cubes. Cook on a low flame for 5 minutes.

6. Enjoy.

Keto Dinner

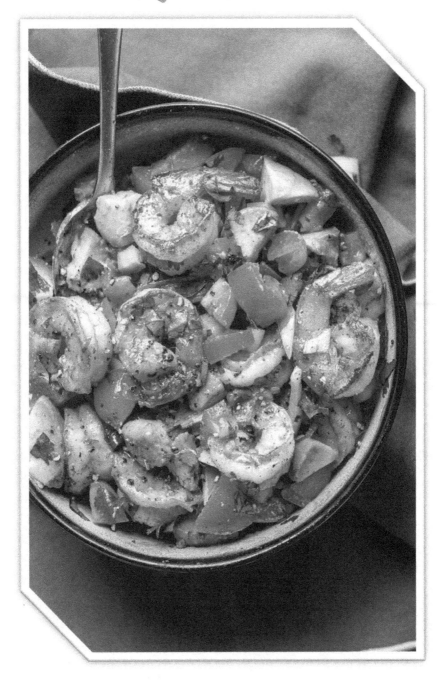

1. Ham-Stuffed Chicken Meatball

Ingredients

- ❖ 1/4 cup chopped ham, fried
- ❖ 2 cups ground chicken
- ❖ 2 tablespoon butter
- ❖ 1 tablespoon onion powder
- ❖ 1 teaspoon garlic powder
- ❖ 1 teaspoon ginger powder
- ❖ Salt to taste
- ❖ 1 teaspoon pepper
- ❖ 1 egg white
- ❖ ¼ cup almond flour

Instructions

1. Add ground chicken, egg white, almond flour, salt, pepper, onion powder, ginger powder, garlic powder, and butter into a food processor. Mix perfectly.

2. Take 1 tablespoon chicken mixture. Make a Pattie into your hand. Place 1 teaspoon ham in the middle. Make a chicken meatball. Do the same with the remaining chicken and ham.

3. Steam the chicken meatballs in a steamer.

4. Serve.

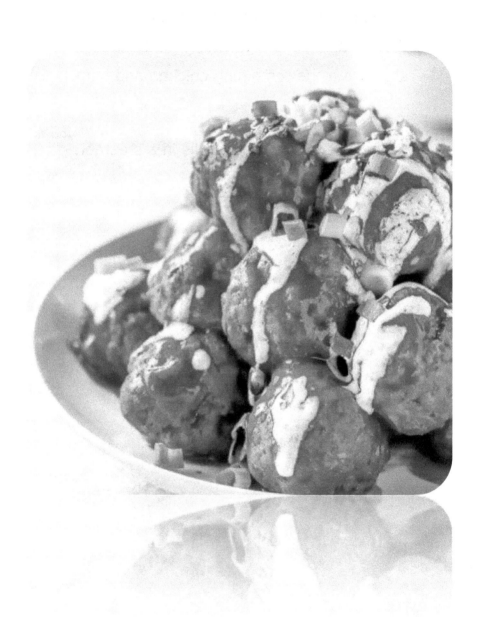

2. Sweet & Sour Prawn

Ingredients

- ❖ 12 prawns
- ❖ 2 tablespoon butter
- ❖ Salt to taste
- ❖ 1 teaspoon pepper
- ❖ 2 tablespoon onion paste
- ❖ 1 teaspoon ginger-garlic paste
- ❖ ½ teaspoon red chili powder
- ❖ 4 tablespoon unsweetened tomato sauce
- ❖ 1 teaspoon soy sauce
- ❖ ½ teaspoon stevia
- ❖ ½ teaspoon oregano

Instructions

1. Melt butter into a frying pan. Add prawns. Sprinkle salt and pepper. Fry for 5 minutes. Take them out.

2. Add onion paste, ginger-garlic paste, and red chili powder into the remaining butter. Sautee for 3 minutes.

3. Now add tomato sauce, stevia, soy sauce, and oregano. Let it come to a boil.

4. Add the prawns. Cook on a medium flame for 5 minutes.

5. Serve.

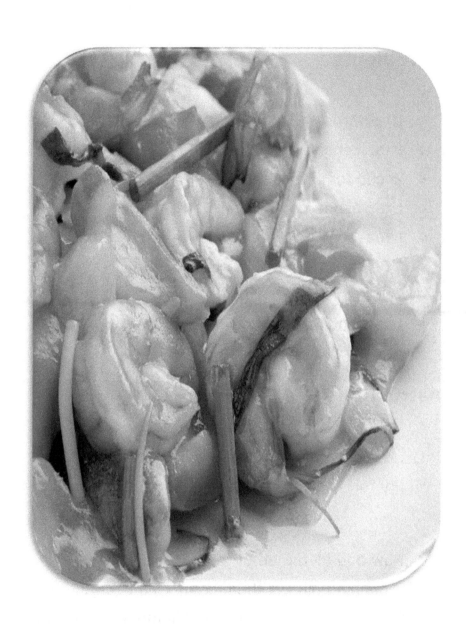

3. Prawn in Tomato Gravy

Ingredients

- ❖ 10 prawns
- ❖ 1 tablespoon avocado oil
- ❖ ½ cup tomato paste
- ❖ 1 tablespoon onion paste
- ❖ 1 teaspoon garlic paste
- ❖ 1 teaspoon red chili powder
- ❖ Salt as needed
- ❖ 1 teaspoon cumin powder

Instructions

1. Heat oil into a frying pan. Add prawn and salt. Fry for 4 to 5 minutes. Take them away.

2. Now add all the other ingredients into the remaining oil. Let them come to a boil. Add the fried prawns. Cook on a low flame for 5 minutes.

3. Serve.

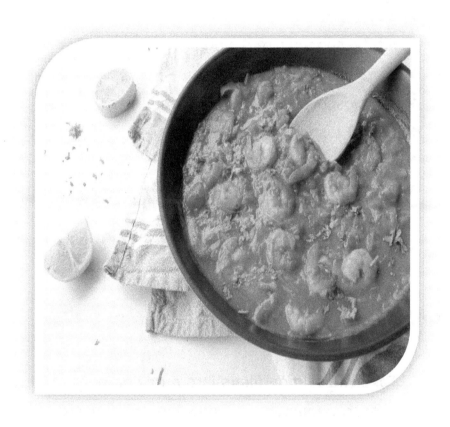

4. Pan-Fried Yogurt Salmon

Ingredients

- ❖ 5 salmon fillets
- ❖ 5 tablespoons Greek yogurt
- ❖ 1 teaspoon onion paste
- ❖ 2 tablespoon ginger-garlic paste
- ❖ Salt to taste
- ❖ 1 teaspoon pepper
- ❖ 1 teaspoon cumin powder
- ❖ 1 tablespoon chopped cilantro
- ❖ 3 tablespoons extra-virgin olive oil

Instructions

1. Take the salmon fillets into a mixing bowl. Add yogurt, pepper, cumin powder, onion paste, ginger-garlic paste, and chopped cilantro. Rub nicely. Put it in the freezer for 20 minutes.

2. Heat the extra-virgin olive oil into a skillet. Place the marinated salmon fillets onto the skillet. Cook on a medium flame for 5 minutes. Then flip the salmon fillets and cook for another 3 minutes on a medium flame.

3. Serve.

5. Okra & Pepper Stir-Fry

Ingredients

- ❖ 1 cup sliced okra
- ❖ ¼ cup finely sliced green bell pepper
- ❖ ¼ cup finely sliced red bell pepper
- ❖ ¼ cup finely sliced yellow bell pepper
- ❖ 2 large onion, finely sliced
- ❖ 1 teaspoon minced garlic
- ❖ 1 teaspoon grated ginger
- ❖ Salt to taste
- ❖ 1 teaspoon pepper
- ❖ 1 tablespoon chopped cilantro
- ❖ 2 tablespoons avocado oil

Instructions

1. Heat avocado oil into a large oak. Add onion, garlic, and ginger. Fry for 3 minutes.

2. Now add sliced okra, sliced red bell pepper, green bell pepper, and yellow bell pepper.

Sprinkle salt, pepper, and chopped cilantro. Fry on a medium flame for 10 minutes. Stir continuously.

3. Serve.

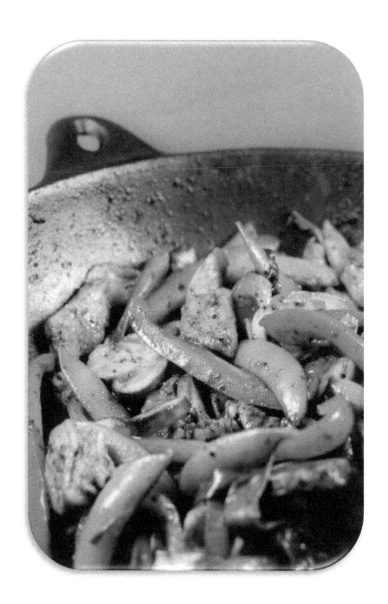

6. Chicken Pattie

Ingredients

- ❖ 1 cup of ground chicken
- ❖ 2 tablespoon almond flour
- ❖ 1 egg white
- ❖ 1 tablespoon onion paste
- ❖ 2 tablespoon ginger-garlic paste
- ❖ 1 tablespoon tomato paste
- ❖ Salt to taste
- ❖ 1 teaspoon pepper
- ❖ 2 tablespoon butter
- ❖ ¼ cup extra-virgin olive oil

Instructions

1. Take a mixing bowl and add ground chicken, salt, pepper, egg white, almond flour, onion paste, tomato paste, and ginger-garlic paste. Mix well. Create four round patties.

2. Heat butter and olive oil into a frying pan. Place the patties onto the pan and cook for 3 minutes on a medium flame. Flip and cook for another 4 minutes.

3. Serve.

7. Pumpkin in Coconut Gravy

Ingredients

- ❖ 1 cup pumpkin, cut into cubes
- ❖ 2 tablespoons butter
- ❖ 2 tablespoon onion paste
- ❖ 2 tablespoon ginger-garlic paste
- ❖ 1 teaspoon red chili powder
- ❖ ½ teaspoon turmeric powder
- ❖ 1 teaspoon pepper
- ❖ Salt to taste
- ❖ 1 tablespoon almond paste
- ❖ 1 cup of coconut milk

Instructions

1. Melt butter into a saucepan. Add onion paste, ginger-garlic paste, red chili powder, cumin powder, almond paste, and turmeric powder. Cook for 3 minutes.

2. Now add the pumpkin cubes. Sprinkle salt and pepper. Sautee for 5 minutes.

3. Then add the coconut milk. Cook for 10 minutes on a low flame.

4. Serve.

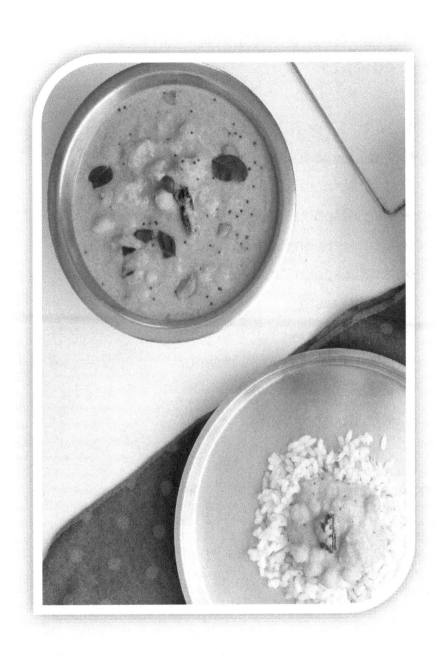

8. Thai Prawn Curry

Ingredients

- ❖ 10 to 12 prawn
- ❖ 2 tablespoon butter
- ❖ 2 tablespoon onion paste
- ❖ 2 tablespoon ginger-garlic paste
- ❖ 1 tablespoon tomato paste
- ❖ 2 tablespoon Thai curry paste
- ❖ Salt to taste
- ❖ 1 teaspoon turmeric powder
- ❖ 1 teaspoon red chili powder
- ❖ ½ teaspoon stevia
- ❖ 1 cup coconut milk

Instructions

1. Melt butter into a saucepan. Add Prawns and salt. Fry for 4 minutes. Take them away.

2. Add onion paste, ginger-garlic paste, tomato paste, turmeric powder, red chili powder, salt,

and stevia into the remaining butter. Cook for two minutes.

3. Now add the coconut milk. Let it come to a boil. Add fried prawns and cook on a low flame for 10 minutes.

4. Serve.

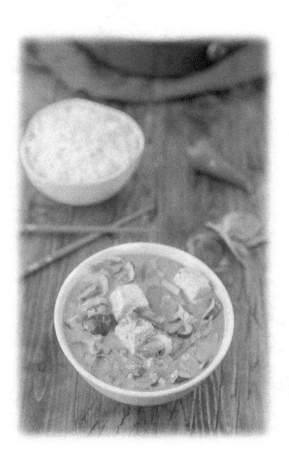

Keto Dessert

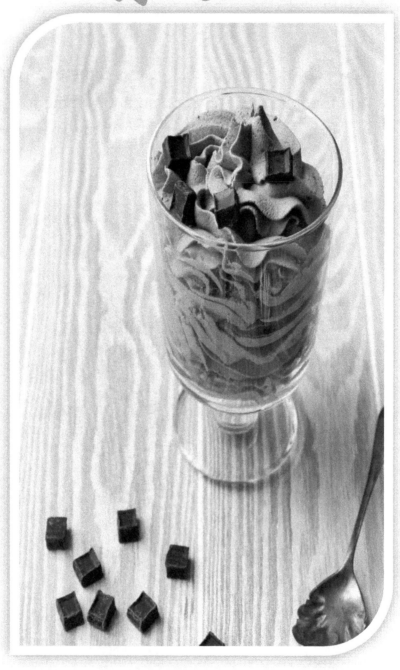

1. Yogurt Strawberry Milk Shake

Ingredients

- ❖ 1 cup strawberries
- ❖ 1 cup thick Greek yogurt
- ❖ ½ almond milk
- ❖ 2 tablespoons stevia
- ❖ ½ teaspoon vanilla extract

Instructions

1. Add everything into a blender. Mix carefully.

2. Serve chilled.

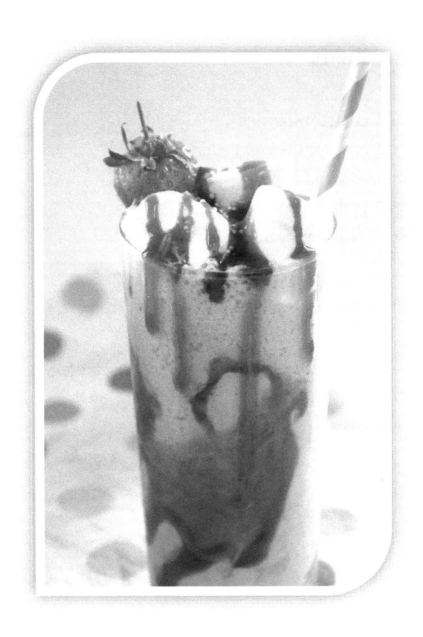

2. Pomegranate Milk Shake

Ingredients

- ❖ 1 cup of pomegranate juice
- ❖ 1 cup coconut milk
- ❖ 1 tablespoon stevia
- ❖ ½ teaspoon vanilla extract
- ❖ ¼ cup heavy cream

Instructions

1. Take a blender and add all the ingredients. Blend smoothly.

2. Serve.

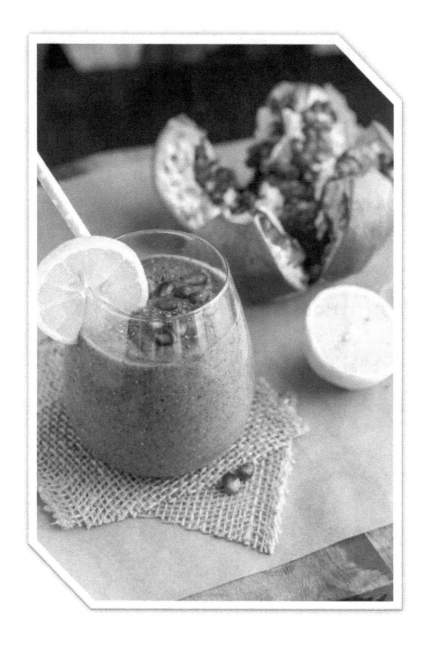

3. Almond mug cake

Ingredients

- ❖ 1 egg
- ❖ 5 tablespoon almond flour
- ❖ 3 tablespoon stevia
- ❖ 2 tablespoon almond milk
- ❖ ½ teaspoon vanilla extract
- ❖ ¼ teaspoon baking powder
- ❖ 2 tablespoon almond butter
- ❖ 1 tablespoon chopped almonds

Instructions

1. Take everything in a mug. Mix smoothly.

2. Microwave for 2 to 4 minutes depending on your microwave type.

3. Enjoy.

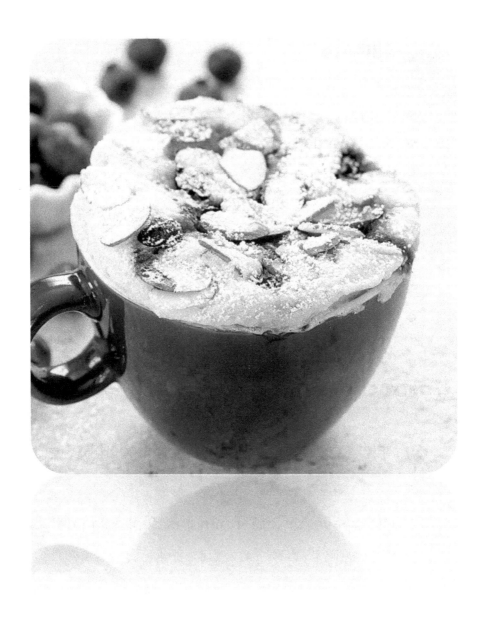

4. Apple Brownie

Ingredients

- ❖ 1 cup grated apple
- ❖ ½ cup melted butter
- ❖ 4 tablespoons cocoa powder
- ❖ 1 tablespoon monk fruit sweetener
- ❖ 1 egg
- ❖ ¼ cup almond flour

Instructions

1. Take a food processor and add all the ingredients. Mix properly.

2. Preheat the oven to 350F. Lightly grease a brownie pan.

3. Pour the batter into the brownie pan. Bake for 20 minutes.

4. Enjoy.

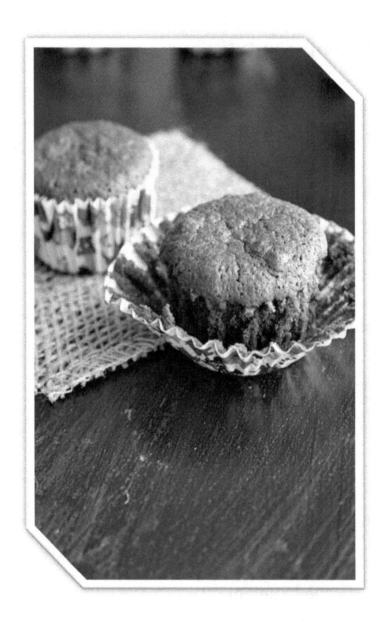

5. Instant Strawberry Ice-cream

Ingredients

- ❖ 1 cup frozen strawberries
- ❖ ½ cup heavy cream, chilled
- ❖ ½ cup cream cheese, chilled
- ❖ ¼ cup Greek yogurt

Instructions

1. Take frozen strawberries, Greek yogurt, cream cheese, and heavy cream into a blender. Blend smoothly. Keep in the fridge for 4 hours.

2. Enjoy.

6. Keto Bottle Gourd Rice Pudding

Ingredients

- ❖ ½ cup grated bottle gourd
- ❖ ¼ cup grated cauliflower
- ❖ 2 cups of almond milk
- ❖ 3 tablespoons erythritol
- ❖ 1 pinch cardamom powder

Instructions

1. Add all the ingredients into a large saucepan. Cook on low flame until you get a thick consistency. You will probably need 10 to 15 minutes. Stir continuously. Otherwise, it will burn at the bottom.

2. Serve cold.

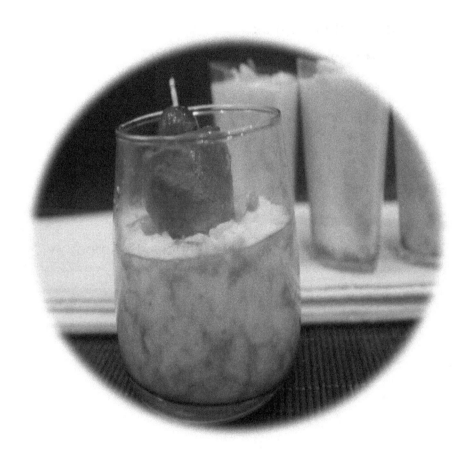

7. Almond Choco Butter Shake

Ingredients

- ❖ 2 cups of almond milk
- ❖ 2 tablespoon almond butter
- ❖ 1 tablespoon stevia
- ❖ 2 tablespoon unsweetened cocoa powder

Instructions

1. Take every ingredient in a blender. Mix smoothly.

2. Serve cold.

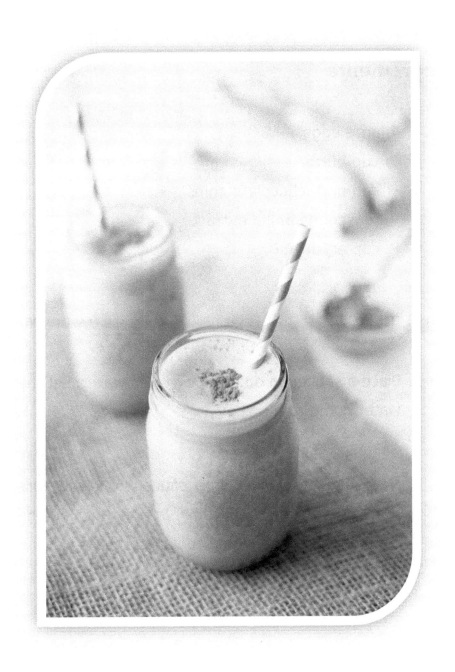

8. Dark Chocolate Curd

Ingredients

- ❖ 4 large eggs
- ❖ ½ cup butter
- ❖ ¼ cup dark chocolate chips
- ❖ ½ teaspoon vanilla extract
- ❖ ½ cup erythritol

Instructions

1. Place a saucepan on the stove with water. Let the water come to a boil.

2. Now place a bowl on the saucepan. Make sure that the bottom of the bowl is not touching the boiling water. The whole cooking process will run with the steam of boiling water.

3. Add eggs, erythritol, dark chocolate chips, and vanilla extract into the bowl. Whisk continuously until the mixer thickens.

4. Now remove the bowl from the heat. Slowly add butter and mix.

5. Enjoy.

Keto Snacks

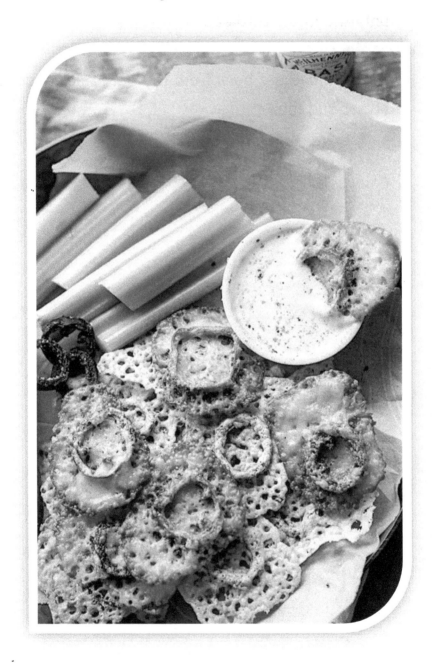

1. Keto Mint Lemonade

Ingredients

* 2 cups water, chilled
* 4 tablespoons lemon juice
* 2 teaspoon stevia
* 2 tablespoons chopped mint leaves.

Instructions

1. Mix all the ingredients.

2. Serve with ice.

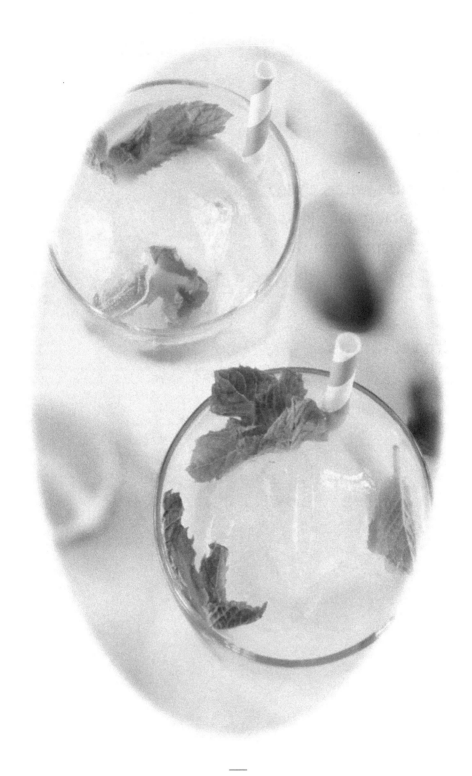

2. Keto Fried Salmon

Ingredients

- 8 salmon fillets
- 1 egg
- ¼ cup heavy cream
- 1 tablespoon onion paste
- 1 tablespoon ginger-garlic paste
- Salt to taste
- 1 teaspoon pepper
- 1 cup almond flour
- 1 cup of grated parmesan cheese
- 1 teaspoon paprika
- 1 teaspoon pink salt
- Sunflower oil for deep frying

Instructions

1. Take a mixing bowl and add egg, heavy cream, salt, pepper, onion paste, and ginger-garlic paste. Mix well. Add the salmon fillets and marinate for 15 minutes.

2. In another mixing bowl add almond flour, parmesan cheese, paprika, and pink salt. Mix well.

3. Now take the marinated salmon fillets and add to the almond flour mix. Coat properly.

4. Heat the oil into a frying pan. Deep fry the salmon fillets on a medium flame until they become golden brown.

5. Enjoy.

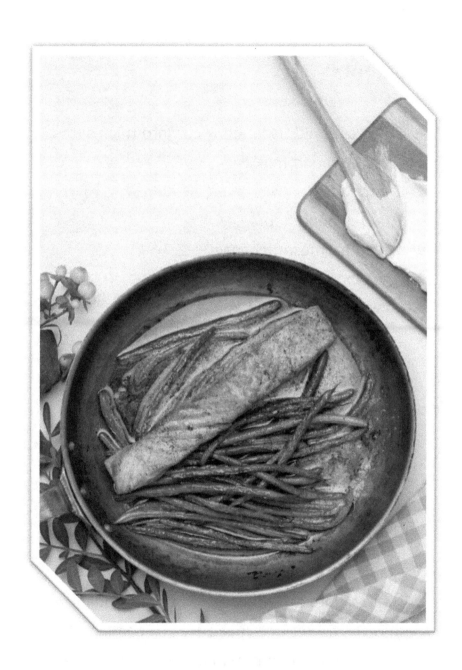

3. Batter Fried Squid

Ingredients

- ❖ 1 cup of squid, cleaned & cut into thick slices
- ❖ ½ cup almond milk
- ❖ 1 large egg
- ❖ 1 cup almond flour
- ❖ ½ cup parmesan cheese
- ❖ 1 teaspoon pink salt
- ❖ 1 teaspoon pepper
- ❖ Sunflower oil for deep frying

Instructions

1. Take a mixing bowl and add almond milk, egg, almond flour, parmesan cheese, pink salt, and pepper. Mix properly.

2. Heat oil into a frying pan. Deep the squid rings into the batter and make a thick coating. Fry in the oil on a medium flame until golden brown.

3. Serve.

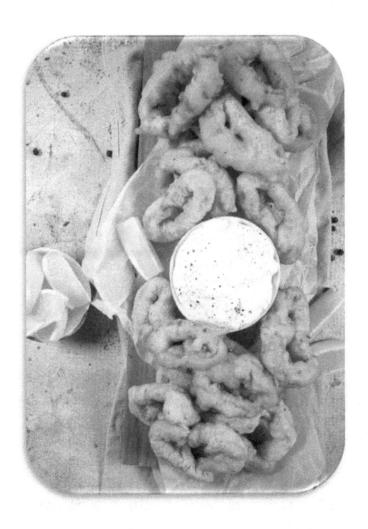

4. Keto Radish Salad

Ingredients

- ❖ 2 radishes, cut into cubes
- ❖ Salt to taste
- ❖ 1 teaspoon pepper
- ❖ 1 tablespoon olive oil
- ❖ ½ cup mayonnaise
- ❖ ½ teaspoon black salt
- ❖ 1 teaspoon chili flakes
- ❖ 1 tablespoon lemon juice

Instructions

1. Preheat the oven to 350F. Place a parchment paper onto a baking tray.

2. Place the radish cubes onto the baking tray. Sprinkle salt, pepper, and olive oil. Bake for 15 minutes.

3. In a mixing bowl add mayonnaise, black salt, chili flakes, and lemon juice. Mix well.

4. Add the roasted radish cubes. Fold gently.

5. Serve.

5. Cauliflower Chips

Ingredients

- ❖ 1 cup grated cauliflower
- ❖ 1 cup cheddar cheese, grated
- ❖ 1 cup grated parmesan cheese
- ❖ Salt to taste
- ❖ 1 teaspoon pepper

Instructions

1. Preheat the oven to 400F. Line a baking tray with parchment paper.

2. Take everything in a bowl and mix well.

3. Make 12 to 15 small balls and place them onto the baking tray. Flatten with the help of your hand.

4. Bake for 15 minutes. Enjoy immediately.

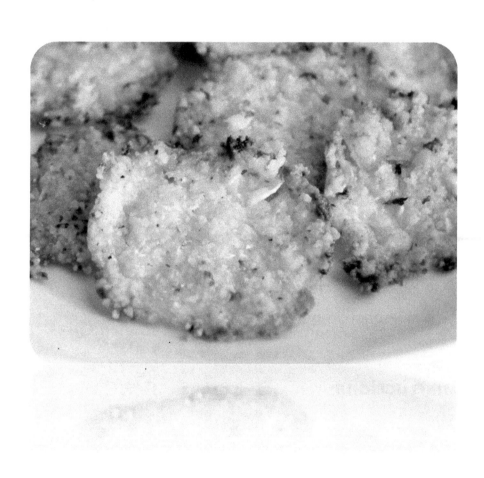

6. Egg & kale salad

Ingredients

- ❖ 2 boiled eggs, cut into cubes
- ❖ ¼ cup chopped & boiled kale
- ❖ ¼ cup chopped avocado
- ❖ ¼ cup chopped romaine lettuce
- ❖ 3 tablespoon extra-virgin olive oil
- ❖ 1 tablespoon apple cider vinegar
- ❖ 2 tablespoon lime juice
- ❖ Salt to taste
- ❖ Pepper to taste
- ❖ 1 teaspoon minced garlic

Instructions

1. In a small bowl add olive oil, apple cider vinegar, lime juice, salt, minced garlic, and pepper. Mix well with the help of a fork.

2. Add eggs, kale, avocado, and lettuce in a salad
   bowl. Pour the salad dressing. Toss gently.

3. Enjoy.

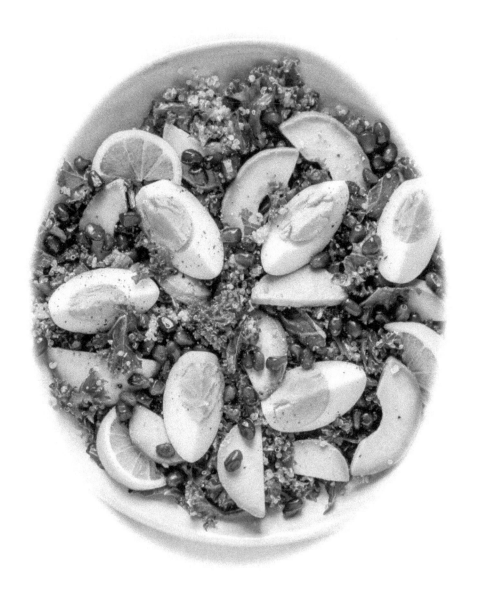

7. Bacon Avocado Devil Egg

Ingredients

- ❖ 8 hard-boiled eggs
- ❖ 2 bacon slices, cooked and crumbled
- ❖ 1 avocado
- ❖ 1 tablespoon lime juice
- ❖ Salt to taste
- ❖ ¼ cup mayonnaise
- ❖ 1 teaspoon paprika

Instructions

1. Cut the boiled eggs in half lengthwise. Take out the yolks and put them into a food processor.

2. Add Avocado, salt, paprika, lime juice, and mayonnaise. Make a fine paste. Add bacon pieces and fold gently.

3. Scoop one dollop of the egg yolk mix into one egg white piece. Do the same with the remaining egg white pieces.

4. Serve.

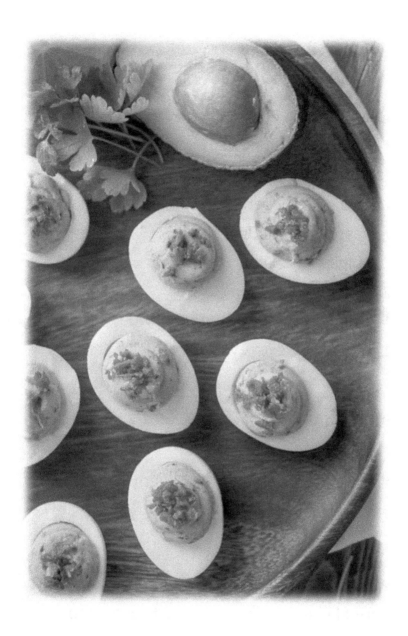

8. Broccoli Hummus

Ingredients

- ❖ 1 cup broccoli florets
- ❖ 1 tablespoon sunflower oil
- ❖ 1 teaspoon sea salt
- ❖ 1 teaspoon pepper
- ❖ 1 teaspoon cumin powder
- ❖ 2 tablespoons tahini
- ❖ 2 tablespoons lemon juice
- ❖ 1 teaspoon smoked paprika powder
- ❖ 1 tablespoon extra-virgin olive oil

Instructions

1. Preheat the oven to 400F. Lightly grease a baking tray.

2. Place the broccoli florets onto the baking tray. Sprinkle sunflower oil, sea salt, and pepper. Bake for 15 minutes.

3. Add roasted broccoli florets into a food processor. Add cumin powder, tahini, lemon juice, smoked paprika powder, and extra-virgin olive oil. Blend smoothly.

4. Serve.

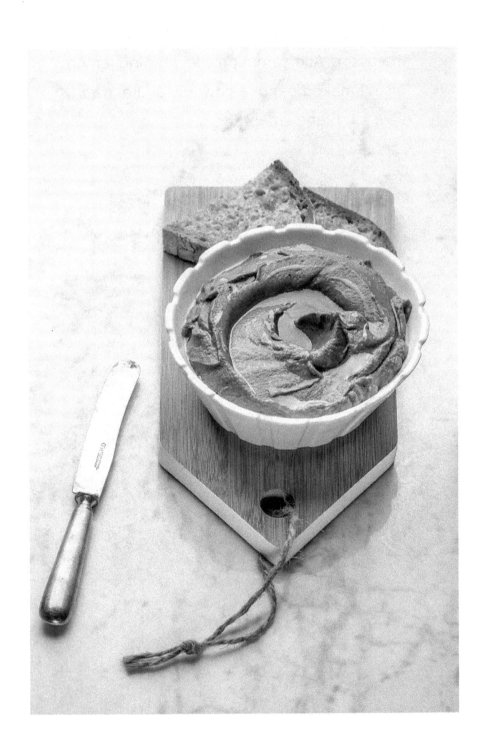

CPSIA information can be obtained
at www.ICGtesting.com
Printed in the USA
BVHW080730140521
607270BV00005B/909

9 781914 121425